EGGS

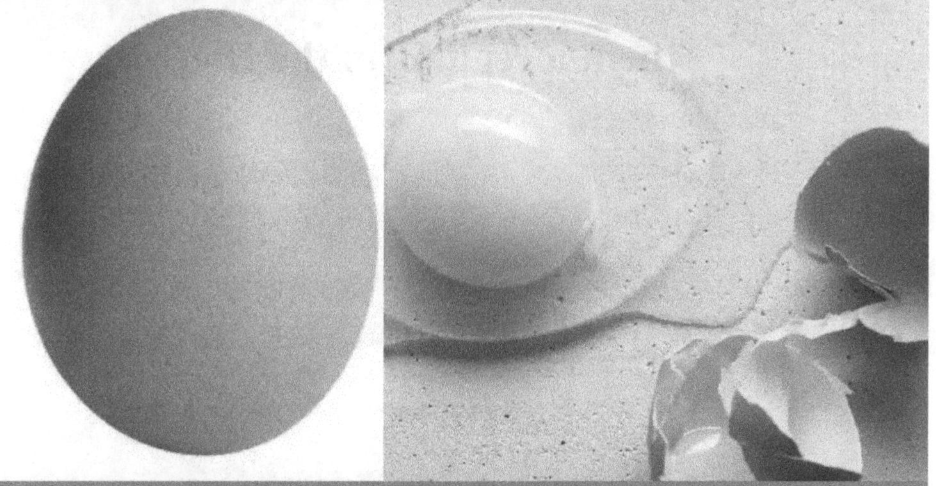

Ignoring the Cholesterol Myth and making them a regular in the Diet

Leslie W. Kings

EGGS

Ignoring the Cholesterol Myth and making them a regular in the Diet

LESLIE W. KINGS

TABLE OF CONTENTS

LIST OF ABBREVIATIONS

- RDA- Recommended Dietary Allowances
- LDL- Low Density Lipoprotein
- HDL- High Density Lipoprotein
- DNA- Deoxyribonucleic acid
- RNA- Ribonucleic acid
- Kcal- Kilocalories (also known as calories)
- mg- Milligram

LIST OF TABLES

LIST OF DIAGRAMS

INTRODUCTION

Eggs are highly nutritious and excellent examples of nutrient-dense foods. They are one of the cheapest sources of protein. Eggs have been a food of much controversy because of their high cholesterol content. Apart from their high cholesterol content, they are also excellent sources of other essential nutrients such as protein, fats, vitamins A and D, choline, phosphorus, riboflavin (vitamin B2), folate (vitamin B9), pantothenic acid (vitamin B5) and cobalamin (vitamin B12). So, avoiding or eliminating eggs from the diet because of their high cholesterol level can cause more harm than good as the body is deprived of other essential and readily available nutrients that can be gotten from them. The average weight of standard-sized eggs is 50g (shell exclusive). In the context of this book, a jumbo or large-sized egg measurement (100g) is used. The reason is the fact that large-sized eggs are preferably demanded by consumers due to their better price-to-size ratio compared to small-sized and standard-sized eggs.

Recent studies and research have shown that dietary cholesterol itself has little or no impact on the increase in blood cholesterol levels. Rather, the type of fats we consume (trans and saturated fats) have a direct impact on the increase in blood cholesterol levels. An increased blood cholesterol level may lead to coronary heart diseases such as atherosclerosis. Eggs meet the dietary guideline for the prevention of heart diseases as they may be high in dietary cholesterol but are low in saturated fat.

STRUCTURE OF AN EGG

1. ALBUMEN: This is also known as the egg white. It is the water and protein store for the developing embryos in eggs. They are high in protein, and low in calories, fats, and cholesterol. These make them a reliable food in a weight loss diet. Egg white plays the primary roles of protection of the yolk and provision of additional nutrition during embryo growth. About 90% of the albumen's composition is water, with dissolved proteins (including albumins, mucoproteins, and globulins) making up the remaining 10%. Egg white has many uses in foods and many other applications, including the preparation of vaccines, such as those for influenza.
2. YOLK: This is the lipid (fats and cholesterol), minerals, vitamins (A, D, and E), and choline store. They are a good source of omega-3 fats as well as folate (vitamin B9), riboflavin (vitamin B2) and cobalamin (vitamin B12).
3. SHELL: This is the thick and strong protective outer layer of eggs. It protects the inner layer of the eggs. It is rich in calcium.

EGGS

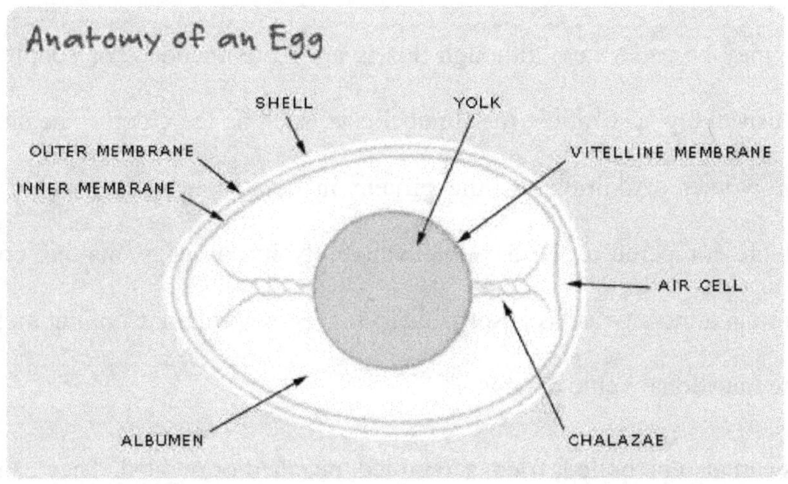

Anatomy of an Egg

MODES OF CONSUMPTION OF EGGS

Eggs may be eaten raw, although this is not recommended for people who may be especially susceptible to salmonellosis, such as the elderly, the sick, or pregnant women. Additionally, the protein in cooked eggs is roughly 91% bioavailable compared to the 51% bioavailability in raw eggs, making cooked eggs' protein almost twice as absorbable as raw eggs' protein. Cooking methods affect the nutritional value of eggs.

Eggs can also be boiled, fried, scrambled, poached or pickled. They can also be used as ingredients in baking. They are used in the food production industry as emulsifiers (to maintain oil in water emulsion) and as thickeners. Every part of an egg can be eaten. The eggshells may not be consumed directly but are a rich store of the mineral calcium which is necessary for bone health, growth and development. The rich calcium content of eggs is exploited by grinding the shells and using them as food additives.

Consumption of raw eggs has been associated with salmonella pathogen which causes salmonellosis, and it is therefore not advisable. Eggs should be properly and thoroughly cooked. Eggs need to be handled and prepared with care to ensure their microbiological safety. Storage conditions should be under a cool and dry environment or by refrigeration if possible.

METHOD OF GRADING EGGS

The most common method of assessing the quality of eggs is by candling. In general, the fresher the egg the higher the quality. Eggs are candled to determine the condition of the air cell, yolk and albumen.

Candling is a method used in embryology to study the growth and development of an embryo inside an egg. This method uses a bright light source behind the larger end of an egg to show details through the shell and is so called because the original sources of light used were candles. Candling is done in a darkened room with the egg held against the light. The light penetrates the egg making it possible to observe the interior part of the egg.

In candling, the egg is held in a slanting position with the larger end of the egg against the hole of the candler. The egg is grasped by the small end and, while held between the thumbs and the tips of the first two fingers, is turned quickly to the right or the left. This moves the contents of the egg and throws the yolk nearer to the shell. Due to the colour of their shells, brown eggs are more difficult to candle compared to white eggs.

The technique of using light to examine eggs is used in the egg production industry to assess the quality of the edible eggs. Eggs are graded according to the size of their air cell, measured during candling. The air cell is situated at the larger end of eggs. A very fresh egg has a small air cell and receives a grade of AA. As the size of the air cell increases and the quality of the egg decreases, the grade moves from AA to A to B. This provides a way of testing the age of an egg: as the air cell increases in size due to air being drawn through pores in the shell as water is lost, the egg becomes less dense.

Another effective way of grading eggs before use in cooking and baking is by placing them in a bowl of warm water. Good eggs remain at the bottom of

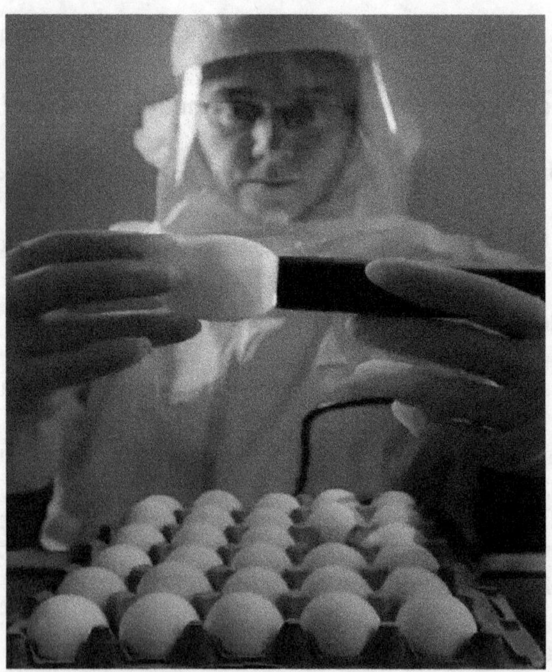

the water while the spoilt or stale eggs float to the surface of the water.

Candling of Eggs

NUTRITIONAL VALUE OF EGGS

Eggs are highly nutritious foods. They may not be the richest in term of caloric content but they are nutrient-dense. A nutrient-dense food is one that provides a relatively high proportion of a person's daily need of essential nutrients while supplying only a small proportion of the daily calories need. The average weight of a standard-sized egg is 50g (shell exclusive). A large-sized egg weighs 100g (shell exclusive) in average.

Nutrient	**Average Amount**
Water	75.8g
Energy	143 kcal
Protein	12.4g
Total Lipids (Fats)	9.96g
Saturated Fatty Acids	3.2g
Monounsaturated Fatty Acids	3.63g
Polyunsaturated Fatty Acids	1.82g
Cholesterol	411mg
Carbohydrates	1.12g
Nitrogen (N)	1.99mg
Calcium (Ca)	48mg
Iron (Fe)	1.67mg

EGGS

Magnesium (Mg)	11.4g
Phosphorus (P)	184mg
Potassium (K)	132mg
Sodium (Na)	129mg
Zinc (Zn)	1.24mg
Copper (Cu)	< 0.1mg
Manganese (Mn)	< 0.05mg
Iodine (I)	49.1 micrograms
Selenium (Se)	31.1 micrograms
Thiamine (Vitamin B1)	0.077mg
Riboflavin (Vitamin B2)	0.419mg
Niacin (Vitamin B3)	< 0.2mg
Pantothenic acid (Vitamin B5)	1.4mg
Vitamin B6	0.063mg
Folate (Vitamin B9)	71 micrograms
Choline	335mg
Cobalamin (Vitamin B12)	1.02 micrograms
Vitamin A	180 micrograms
Vitamin D	2.46 micrograms 98.4 IU
Lutein	230 micrograms

EGGS

Zeaxanthin	229 micrograms

Nutritional Value per 100g of Eggs

A 100g egg supplies 143 kcal of energy of which about 63% is from its high fat content. The protein and carbohydrate content provide about 35% and 0.031% respectively of the total calories in eggs. A point of note is that 1g of fat translates to 9 kcal of energy while 1g each of protein and carbohydrate translates to 4 kcal each of energy.

Eggs have low carbohydrate content. The egg white (albumen) is high in protein and contains 75.8g of water. Egg protein like other animal proteins is of high biological value as it contains all essential amino acids in decent proportions. The egg yolk is rich in fat and has a very high cholesterol content.

Egg raises the body levels of both low-density lipoprotein (bad cholesterol) and high-density lipoprotein (good cholesterol). The American Heart Association sets the RDA for cholesterol at less than 300mg per day. The body also synthesizes its cholesterol from the fats, sugars and protein ingested from the diet. 75% of body cholesterol is biosynthesized in the liver. The remaining 25% is gotten from diet. Recent studies and research have shown that dietary cholesterol itself isn't as harmful as exaggerated and may not contribute to the increase in blood cholesterol levels. Rather, dietary saturated fat should be limited to not more than 10% of the total calorie intake level of an individual, and trans fat (man-made fat) should be avoided. These two types of fats have been shown to increase LDL concentration in the body. This can be harmful as an increased LDL to HDL ratio may lead to increased direct transportation of cholesterol through the arteries thereby clogging the arteries. This leads to atherosclerosis, a coronary heart disease. High level of HDL in the blood compared to LDL is recommended as HDL (good cholesterol) carries cholesterol back to the liver where they are stored and released in times of need. HDL also helps in carrying clogged LDL cholesterol in the arteries back to the liver where they are broken down into individual components and released or excreted from the body. Cholesterol is a natural substance that is produced in the liver and is also found in animal-based foods. It is a waxy, fatty substance that travels through the bloodstream. Cholesterol is essential in building cells and in the production of certain hormones (e.g. oestrogen, cortisone and testosterone) as well as bile acid which plays a crucial role in fat digestion. It is also a precursor for vitamin D3 (cholecalciferol). In the case where dietary cholesterol is higher than normal, the body synthesizes less of it to create a balance in the body. This compensatory mechanism is one key reason why dietary cholesterol has little or no effect on blood cholesterol level. Apart from increased weight gain and possibly obesity, high cholesterol and lipid content in the body isn't as harmful except they find themselves in high concentrations in unwanted areas and tissues such as the blood and blood vessels. This is only made possible by the action of LDL fat transporter.

EGGS

Eggs are excellent sources of cobalamin (vitamin B12). A large-sized egg supplies 1.02 micrograms of vitamin B12. The RDA for vitamin B12 (according to the National Research Council {1989}) is 2 micrograms/day. That is to say that a large-sized egg in our daily diet is enough to cover 50% of the body's vitamin B12 daily needs. Cobalamin is essential in the production of red blood cells, haemoglobin, hormones and DNA in the body. It also prevents megaloblastic anaemia, an ailment where the red blood cells become larger than normal. It is also good for healthy eyes, brain, heart, hair, skin and nails.

Egg yolks are good sources of vitamin D. A large-sized egg supplies 2.46 micrograms of vitamin D. That is about 16.4% of the body's RDA. The RDA for vitamin D is 15 micrograms per day (National Institutes of Health, 2022). The remaining percentage can be got from other food sources in the diet. Vitamin D obtained from eggs is biologically inert and must undergo two hydroxylation reactions in the body for activation. The first hydroxylation, which occurs in the liver, converts vitamin D3 (cholecalciferol) into 25-hydroxyvitamin D [25(OH)D], also known as calcifediol. The second hydroxylation reaction takes place in the kidney where the calcifediol is converted to 1,25-hydroxyvitamin D [1,25(OH)2D], also known as calcitriol. Calcitriol is the physiologically active form of vitamin D3. It travels through the body, affecting almost every cell. The form of vitamin D present in eggs is Vitamin D3 (cholecalciferol). Vitamin D is essential for the regulation of the absorption of calcium and phosphorus, which are essential for the healthy growth and development of bones and teeth. Vitamin D also plays a role in immune functions. Deficiency of vitamin D results in rickets, a disease in children where the bone tissues are poorly mineralized resulting in soft, weak and skeletally deformed bones.

Egg yolks are good sources of folate (vitamin B9). The RDA for folate is 400 micrograms per day (National Institutes of Health, 2021). A large-sized egg has a folate supply of 71 micrograms which is about 17.8% of the RDA. Folate plays a role in cell division and growth. It is involved in the synthesis of RNA and DNA. This explains why it is a very important nutrient during pregnancy. The RDA for folate increases with increased demands during pregnancy. The RDA for folate rises to as much as 600 micrograms per day during pregnancy. This is due to the continuous supply of blood to the developing foetus. Folate is also essential in the production of healthy red blood cells. Low intake of folate may lead to megaloblastic anaemia, poor immune function and poor digestion.

Eggs are good sources of phosphorus. The RDA of phosphorus is 700 mg/day (National Institutes of Health, 2021). A large-sized egg provides 184mg of phosphorus which makes up for 26.3% of the daily requirement value. Phosphorus is essential for bone and teeth formation, growth and development. It makes up cell membrane structure and is also essential for body metabolism such as energy production, nerve conduction and maintenance of cellular functions. It also contributes to DNA and RNA formation and is responsible for the storage and transmission of genetic information.

Egg yolk is an excellent source of vitamin A. Vitamin A is a fat-soluble vitamin that plays an important role in vision and eye health, bone and teeth development, hair growth and in reproduction. It also regulates the immune system. The RDA of vitamin A is 1000 micrograms per day in men and 800 micrograms in women. A 100g portion of egg supplies 180 micrograms of vitamin A which accounts for 18% to 22.5% of the daily value. Egg yolk provides vitamin A in the form of preformed vitamin A which is readily absorbed in the body.

Vitamin B2 (riboflavin) is another water-soluble vitamin that is present in abundance in eggs. The vitamin B2 content of large-sized egg is 0.419mg. That covers a sizeable percentage of the RDA of riboflavin which stands at 1.3 mg/day and 1.1mg/day for men and women respectively (Gebhardt and Thomas, 2002). A diet containing a large-sized egg has a 32-38% daily value of vitamin B2. The body can only store a little of the vitamin B2 from the diet, usually in the kidney, heart and liver. Excess is excreted in the urine. Vitamin B2 has to be gotten continually from our diet to serve the vital functions it plays in the body. Vitamin B2 plays roles in the maintenance of healthy red blood cells, energy extraction, skin protection and eye health.

EGGS

Eggs are excellent sources of vitamin B5 (pantothenic acid). A 100g portion of eggs is rich in 1.4mg of vitamin B5. The RDA for vitamin B5 is 5 mg/day (National Institutes of Health, 2021). A diet containing a large egg, therefore, covers 28% of the daily value for the water-soluble micronutrient vitamin B5. The richest source of vitamin B5 is beef liver but eggs also provide an excellent amount of vitamin B5 in the diet. The major function of vitamin B5 is in energy extraction. Vitamin B5 is essential for the synthesis of coenzyme A and acyl protein carrier which are subsequently used for fatty acids synthesis and breakdown. It also functions in the maintenance of cholesterol level by increasing HDL (good cholesterol) and lowering LDL (bad cholesterol) and triglycerides levels in the body. This has an anti-inflammatory effect and helps in preventing coronary heart diseases. This also helps in counterbalancing the high cholesterol content of eggs.

One special nutrient found in abundance in eggs is choline. A large-sized egg supplies 335mg of choline which is about 61% of the daily value. This makes eggs one of the best sources of choline. The RDA for choline is 550mg and 425mg per day for men and women respectively (National Institutes of Health, 2022). Choline is essential in maintaining the structural integrity of cells. Choline can be synthesized by the body but the body still requires extra choline from the diet as that synthesized by the body is not sufficient to meet the daily needs of the body. They are important components of cell membranes in the form of sphingomyelin and phosphatidylcholine. Choline helps in brain and nerve functions as they are needed in the synthesis of the neurotransmitter acetylcholine. It plays important role in modulating gene expression, cell membrane signaling, lipid transport and metabolism and early brain development.

Eggs have a moderate zinc content. A large egg makes up 11-16% of the daily value for zinc. The RDA for zinc is 11 mg/day and 8 mg/day for men and women respectively (National Institutes of Health, 2022). A large-sized egg (100g) in the diet supplies 1.24mg of zinc. Zinc is one very important mineral as it plays a lot of roles in the body. The functions of zinc include immunity and wound healing, maintenance of the senses of smell and taste, reproduction, growth and development. Zinc along with other antioxidants delays the progression of age-related macular degradation and vision loss by preventing cellular damage of the retina.

Eggs are excellent sources of the mineral selenium. A 100g portion of egg contains 31.1 micrograms of selenium. This accounts for 55.54% of the daily value for selenium as its RDA stands at 55 micrograms per day (National Institutes of Health, 2021). Selenium is a constituent of selenoproteins which play critical roles in reproduction, thyroid hormone metabolism, DNA synthesis and protection of body cells from oxidative damage and infection.

SIDE EFFECTS OF EGGS

As with the saying “Too much of anything is bad”, excessive consumption of eggs is bad and may have some side effects.

1. Salmonellosis: This occurs when eggs are eaten raw or not properly cooked.
2. Food Allergy: This applies only to people with a rare allergy to eggs.
3. Type II Diabetes: Eggs are rich in fat, and when taken in excessive amounts like other fat-rich food, it may result in the body developing insulin resistance. This is a precursor to type II diabetes as the body does not respond to the insulin released by the pancreas. This leads to increased concentration of sugar in the blood.
4. Too many eggs in one meal, like other protein-rich foods, may result in bloating, nausea, vomiting, stomach cramp and other stomach disorders.
5. Protein Overload: Eggs have high protein content. Excessive overload of protein may affect the kidneys as it damages the kidneys’ capability to filter toxins from the blood. This could lead to ammonia toxicity in the blood which may lead to death.

RECOMMENDED DIETARY ALLOWANCE FOR EGGS

There is no longer any specific limit on the number of eggs that can be eaten on a daily or weekly basis, but the recommendation to limit dietary cholesterol intake to an average of 300 mg/day still stands. Based on recent studies and research, I would personally recommend 1 egg per day (1 large-sized egg or 2 standard-sized eggs). One major cause for alarm on excessive consumption of eggs is the high cholesterol level. It exceeds the RDA of less than 300mg stipulated by the American Heart Association. But recent studies and research have also allayed this fear based on the conclusion that dietary cholesterol has little or no effect on blood cholesterol level increase. Rather, excessive cholesterol concentration in the blood has been associated with an increased saturated fat intake which is known to subsequently increase LDL cholesterol level (bad cholesterol) in the blood. This is pro-inflammatory and can lead to coronary heart diseases such as atherosclerosis. Atherosclerosis is a type of heart disease where cholesterol clogs the walls of the arteries and reduce the area of blood flow in arteries. This results in increased blood pump pressure to the arteries by the heart. Another point of note is that to maintain a diet of one egg per day, the overall daily cholesterol intake from other foods in the diet should be low.

A justifiable reason to consume eggs regardless of their high cholesterol content is the fact that they are low in saturated fat and total calories.

Exceptions to my recommended one egg per day in the diet are older adults with lower basal metabolic rate and reduced rate of body metabolism. Other exceptions are people suffering from certain disorders that limit the absorption of certain nutrients from diet and people with high blood cholesterol levels who are sensitive to dietary cholesterol intake.

Some nutrients such as vitamin B5 have also been found to counterbalance the effect of high cholesterol in eggs. Vitamin B5 helps in the maintenance of cholesterol level by increasing HDL and lowering LDL and triglyceride levels in the blood.

A common mode of egg consumption is frying. This method more often than not involves the use of about 4 standard-sized eggs or 2 large-sized eggs. This raises a very important question; Is the use of 2 large eggs not too excessive, as it exceeds the daily limit with the largest margin? The answer is having a 2-egg meal can be fine if eaten along with food with low to zero fat content (such as yam, potato, grains or bread) or if the meal is balanced by having a low fat or cholesterol diet the following day (such as cereals, fat-free milk, rice and fruits). In this way, the average cholesterol intake across maybe 7 days still falls not too distant from the recommended 300 mg/day daily limit.

REFERENCES

1. "Candling eggs". (2019). University of Illinois Extension. Retrieved 2012-06-06.
2. "Full Report (All Nutrients): 01123, Eggs, Grade A, Large, egg whole". USDA Branded Food Products Database.
3. https://en.m.wikipedia.org/wiki/Egg_as_food
4. Kathleen Meister. (2002). The Role of Egg in the Diet. *American Council on Science and Health*. New York.
5. Institutes of Medicine. (2005). Dietary Reference Intakes for Energy, Carbohydrates, Fiber, Fat, Fatty Acids, Cholesterol, Protein and Amino Acids/Panel on Macronutrients, Panel on the Definition of Dietary Fiber, Subcommittee on Upper Reference Levels of Nutrients, Subcommittee on Interpretation and Uses of Dietary Reference Intakes, and the Standing Committee on the Scientific Evaluation of Dietary Reference Intakes, Food and Nutrition Board. *The National Academies Press*. Washington DC.
6. National Academy of Sciences. (2004). Dietary Reference Intakes for Water, Potassium, Sodium, and Sulfate. *National Academy Press*. Washington DC.
7. National Institutes of Health. (2021). Folate Fact Sheet for Health Professional.

8. National Institutes of Health. (2021). Pantothenic Acid Fact Sheet for Health Professional.
9. National Institutes of Health. (2021). Phosphorus Fact Sheet for Health Professional.
10. National Institutes of Health. (2021). Selenium Fact Sheet for Health Professional.
11. National Institutes of Health. (2022). Choline Fact Sheet for Health Professional.
12. National Institutes of Health. (2022). Vitamin D Fact Sheet for Health Professional.
13. National Institutes of Health. (2022). Zinc Fact Sheet for Health Professional.
14. National Research Council. (1989). Recommended Dietary Allowances. 10th Edition. *National Academy Press.* Washington DC.
15. Susan, E. Gebhardt and Robin, G. Thomas. (2002). Nutritive Value of Foods. *United States Department of Agriculture, Agricultural Research Service, Home and Garden Bulletin 72*. Maryland.

www.ingramcontent.com/pod-product-compliance
Lightning Source LLC
LaVergne TN
LVHW052115160826
845678LV00015B/3559

* 9 7 9 8 3 6 8 0 4 9 0 2 1 *